Made in United States
North Haven, CT
18 October 2022

25603929R00067